Kicking Cancer in the Butt

A Guide to Thriving In Spite of Anal Cancer

Theresa Mayhew

This book is dedicated to my husband, Hugh, my family and friends, all the people who have cancer (or are in remission), and those who support someone with cancer.

I offer a special thank you to my friends and supporters from Blogforacure.com who contributed their wisdom, stories, and suggestions, especially Martha who makes it a point to befriend and support the newcomers.

Contents

Introduction

This book is about the BIG C.

From my perspective it's called that because if uttered out loud it's certainly a death sentence, or at best it turns your life upside down, inside out, and round and round (as the song goes, but it was referring to something much more pleasant, I'm sure).

Cancer has the ability to make the best of us panic stricken and fearful or it can become the turning point in our lives, helping us to transform into courageous, grateful, and more alive spiritual beings.

Specifically, this book is about the type of cancer I was diagnosed with which is cloacogenic carcinoma; however, many of the ideas and suggestions will apply to the various types of anal and rectal cancer, as well as all other forms of cancer.

The suggestions in this book are from my experience (and those of my online friends from BlogforaCure.com) and what's worked well for us.

I've written the book in three parts - Before, During, and After - so you can jump ahead to whatever stage is applicable to your situation. This book is also written for your friends and family to help them know how to support you (if you're the one with the cancer diagnosis).

PART 1 - BEFORE

Chapter 1: What is Anal Cancer?

Anal cancer is a disease in which malignant (cancer) cells form in the tissues of the anus. According to information found at www.DoctorsLounge.com, "Anal cancer is an uncommon malignancy with an annual incidence of approximately 6 per 1,000,000 and accounting for only a small percentage (4%) of all cancers of the lower gastrointestinal tract. *Anal cancer is not the same as colorectal cancer.*"

Anal cancer affects the most distal 1½ " of the colon called the anus, the muscular sphincter, and anal structures that are outside the colon and are similar to skin tissues.

Fortunately, it is relatively easy to detect in most cases, and there are even tests for people at high risk for anal cancer that can detect signs of the disease before the cancer actually develops. The exact cause of anal cancer is unknown. In many cases, anal cancer is believed to be linked to infection by the human papilloma virus (HPV), the same virus that causes many cases of cervical cancer in women.

Risk Factors

Risk factors include the following:

- Being over 50 years old.
- Being infected with the human papillomavirus (HPV) can affect the risk of developing anal cancer.
- The presence of genital warts increases the risk by a factor of 30.

According to the American Cancer Society, women are slightly more likely to get anal cancer than men; most anal cancer occurs in adults over age 35.

In 2010, an estimated 5,290 adults (2,100 men and 3,190 women) in the United States will be diagnosed with anal cancer. It is estimated that 710 deaths (260 men and 450 women) from this disease will occur this year.

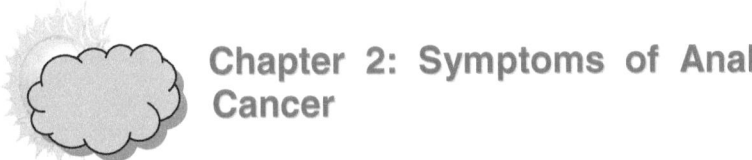# Chapter 2: Symptoms of Anal Cancer

My symptoms included occasional blood in the stool and anal itching. Had I been more aware that these are symptoms of anal cancer I would have gone to the doctor much sooner. As it happens, the tumor was already 3 cm (about 1 ¼"). I don't know if the treatment protocol would have been different and I'm lucky the cancer hadn't spread.

Since getting an early diagnosis is important, go see your doctor if you have any of the following symptoms:

- Pain or pressure in the anal area
- Blood in the stool or from the anal area (I figured I just had hemorrhoids and waited 2 months before seeing my doctor, learn from my experience)
- Itching in the anal area or a discharge
- Any kind of change in your bowel movements (change in shape and frequency)
- A lump or swelling

Some of these symptoms may not seem all that significant. It's not like finding a lump in your breast one day and knowing that it's something really abnormal. Too often people think a little blood in their stool is due to pushing too hard to have a bowel movement or that it's just "a hemorrhoid".

It's a good idea not to self diagnose. Just go and have your doctor check it out and you'll relieve yourself of needless worry (or more importantly find out early enough to have a better chance of surviving an aggressive form of cancer).

If you have any of these symptoms, see your doctor. Not all cases of anal cancer exhibit symptoms, so if you fall into a *high risk category for anal cancer, you may want to schedule annual visits to your doctor and discuss any concerns.

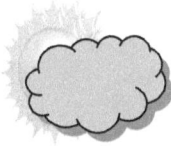 ## Chapter 3: Diagnosis

Types of Anal Cancer

There are different types of cancer of the anus because there are different types of cells in the anus.

Squamous cell carcinomas are the most common type and account for about 70% - 90% of all anal cancers. This type begins in the cells that line the anal margin and most of the anal canal.

Cloacogenic carcinomas (sometimes referred to as basaloid or transitional cell carcinomas) make up about 20% to 25% of all anal cancers.

Adenocarcinomas make up less than 5% of all cases of anal cancer and grow from glandular cells which produce mucus in the anus.

Anal cancer may be discovered during a routine digital rectal exam (DRE), in which a medical professional inserts a gloved finger past the anus to feel for abnormalities. It is also diagnosed with an anal Pap smear, in which a cotton swab is inserted past the anus and swirled to capture a tissue sample

Another test to determine whether you have anal cancer or other problems with the colon is a colonoscopy. A routine Colonoscopy at the age of 50 is recommended by the medical profession.

Questions to ask your doctor

- What kind of anal cancer do I have?

- Has my cancer spread beyond the primary site?

- What is the stage of my cancer? What does the staging mean in my case?

- What treatment choices do I have?

- What treatment would you recommend for me?

- What side effects can I expect from my treatment?

- What are the other risks of treatment?

- How soon after treatment starts will we know if it's working?

- How long will it take me to recover from treatment?

- How soon after treatment can I return to my normal activities, such as work, school, exercise, or sex?

- Will I need to have a colostomy?

- Based on what you've learned about my cancer, what is my outlook?

- What are the chances that my cancer will recur?

- Does one type of treatment reduce the risk of recurrence more than another?

- What should I do to be ready for treatment?

- Should I get a second opinion?

- How long will my treatment, including follow-up, last?

- Will there be permanent issues relating to bowel function?

- Will there be permanent issues relating to sexual function?

- Could this treatment affect my fertility? If so, can you recommend a fertility specialist?

- How will this treatment affect my daily life? Will I be able to work, exercise, and perform my usual activities?

- If I'm worried about managing the costs related to my cancer care, who can help me with these concerns?

- What follow-up tests will I need, and how often will I need them?

- How can I keep myself as healthy as possible during treatment?

- What support services are available to me? To my family?

Write Your Own Questions Here:

 ## Chapter 4: Telling Your Family & Friends

Telling your family and friends may be one of the most challenging parts of this journey. I chose to call my family and friends individually so they heard it from me. I also decided to share my diagnosis and the type of cancer (even though it's really personal) because I wanted others to have the benefit of my experience. If even one person is saved from going through this because they found out early enough, it's worth it to me.

A friend of mine called just after I received the news. I told him about my symptoms and he shared that he was experiencing the same symptoms. Fortunately, he decided that it would be a good idea to schedule an appointment with his doctor and have a colonoscopy. I'm grateful to report that his was clear.

Having a support system will help you immensely during your treatment and recovery. Let them help you. I'm sure you've been on the other side of this fence when someone you love has been ill or in need of help in some way. Doesn't it make you feel better to be able to do something to make them more comfortable? Now it's your turn to receive. Allowing your friends and family to do something for you is a gift to them.

Chapter 5: Preparing for Treatment: Alternative or Traditional?

After the shock wore off (from that announcement, "You have an aggressive form of cancer."), I decided to take all the information on health and healing that I knew about and put it to use.

I really wanted to use natural cures for cancer initially and did a lot of research to find out what worked for other people. In the end, it was the talk with the oncologist and inward direction that convinced me to take the traditional path. I'm still incorporating natural methods to help ease the discomfort of the side effects and will happily share them with you.

I am self-admittedly addicted to sugar and have quit drinking coffee more times than I can count. I also know that having too much acid in my body can lead to health problems. So, one of the first things I did was eliminate all sugar, caffeine, and processed foods. It's not that I was consuming very much of these, but it was something I could do for myself.

Last year I came across a book that explains how to go about changing over to an alkaline diet and all the healthy benefits that go along with it. Everything I've read so far about cancer indicates that this is the best type of eating plan.

To help myself feel less fear and more in control of my circumstances I decided I needed to be proactive and create a healing plan. Here's what it looks like:

- Daily Spiritual Exercises of ECK
- Good nutrition – alkaline diet, herbal extracts, Vitamin D
- Daily physical exercise – walking our dogs, The 5 Rites, resistance
- Healing Codes - a method for reducing stress
- Watching a MindMovie I made with truth focus statements
- Clean the clutter around the house – this step just helps me feel like I'm doing something to help myself

I'd like to be able to say that I've kept up with my plan and most of it I have. Once I decided to go the traditional route of chemo and radiation treatment, some of it went by the wayside. My digestive system doesn't tolerate certain foods and when I was dealing with side effects of the chemo, I just couldn't eat the same way I had planned. I also didn't have the energy for the physical exercise.

The rest of the plan is intact and I am very happy to say that the spiritual exercises, Healing Codes and the MindMovie helped tremendously to keep me from succumbing to anxiety, panic, and fear.

Do whatever works for you to help bring a sense of calm and peace. Some examples are prayer, meditation, spiritual exercises, and yoga.

The mind and imagination will want to take over. Remember that you (Soul) are in charge and control where your mind and imagination wander. If you feel like you're losing control, this might be a good time to rely on your supporters. Call someone and talk about it.

There is also a wonderful web site called www.BlogforaCure.com. It's an online community of people with cancer. The individuals there create their own blogs and write about their experiences with the disease. It is very helpful to hundreds of people and their families. You can find out from someone who's gone through almost every type of cancer and its treatment what to expect.

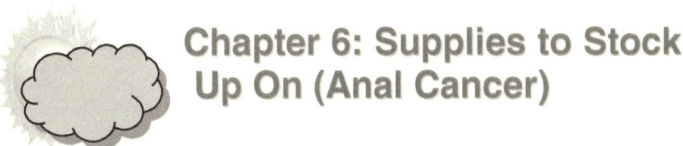

Chapter 6: Supplies to Stock Up On (Anal Cancer)

Having the following list of products on hand before you start treatment will eliminate the last minute efforts when you really need them. Maybe you won't want or need everything on this list, but most of them will have been acquired by the end of your chemo and radiation treatment.

- Aquaphor (available over the counter at the drug store, but it's less expensive on Amazon).

- Pads – sometimes they're called Chux. These are going to come in handy around week 4-5 of radiation so you can lay down on your sofa bare bottomed and not worry about leaving a stain.

- For women – buy underwear 1-2 sizes larger than you normally wear, or plan on borrowing your husband's boxer shorts.

- Flexible/soft ice packs – I applied an ice pack for a minute or so to my bottom (as well as the front) when I had to go to the bathroom. It helped numb the area before I peed or went #2. (The earplugs may come in handy for members of your household; sorry, I don't mean to scare you.)

- Juven - The dietitian suggested that I start drinking a product called Juven. It has HGB, L-Glutamine and L-Arginine and helps promote wound heeling. This was a life saver during the first few weeks. I was able to get by without the pain meds for a little while.

- Ear plugs – I used them to block out the hum of the chemo pump. It goes off every 30 seconds.

- Reynold's Solution – this is a prescription. Ask your oncologist about it. It's to help relieve the mouth sores (thrush) that develop as a result of the chemotherapy.

- Sesame oil – I used sesame oil to swish in my mouth to remove bacteria.

- Donut – this is a special cushion with an indentation in the middle that conforms to body contours reducing pressure point discomfort

- Flex straws – it sure makes it easier to drink from a straw when you're in a reclining position or when your mouth is full of sores and you just want the liquid to go down your throat easier.

- Handheld Shower Spray

- Chlorine Free Baby Wipes

- Squeeze bottle small (for diluting pee)

- Soft toothbrush and toothpaste for sensitive gums

- Biotene rinse and toothpaste

- Panty Liners with wings (or thicker) for diarrhea

- Lots of antibacterial hand sanitizer

- A&D Ointment

- Aloe Vera gel

- Extra towels and sheets

- Disinfectant cleaner like Lysol

- Lip stuff for chapped lips

- Sitz bath (I'd put this at the top of the list!)

- Cotton skirts you can wear to "air out". (This could be a way for your creative friends or family members to do something for you. Let them know they could make you a simple pull-on style skirt to wear instead of sweat pants or pajama bottoms.)

- A few good books and movies.

- Sorbet

- Bread that is not high fiber

- Nut butter

- Soups

- Veggies for juicing (as tolerated – you'll have to see how you do with fresh veggies & fruit)

- Omega 3 oil

- Greens for drinks

- Things you might not normally eat like: organic Mac and Cheese, Jello, popsicles (you can make homemade w/o sugar with a popsicle mold)

- Gatorade

- Baby powder for the genital area. Try it after you've healed from the radiation burns to help keep the skin from sticking together (especially for the guys).

All of the above products are available on Amazon and you can create a wish list. Let your friends or family members know what you need from this list and let them help you out.

 # Chapter 7: Financial Assistance

Dealing with cancer is stressful enough without adding the concerns about how you're going to pay for treatment.

The social worker at your hospital will be able to assist you in finding financial aid if you don't have insurance.

There were several local organizations that have special grants available for cancer patients where I live.

The same may be true for your community and the social worker will have that information available.

PART II - DURING

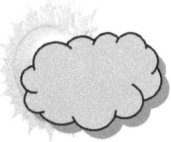 **Chapter 8: Treatment**

The treatment options depend on the stage of the cancer.

There are three basic types of treatment used for anal cancer:

- Radiation therapy – high-dose x-rays to kill cancer cells
- Chemotherapy – giving drugs to kill cancer cells.
- Surgery – an operation to remove the cancer

Combination therapy including radiation therapy and chemotherapy is now considered the standard treatment for most anal cancers. If the tumor does not respond completely to combination therapy, if it recurs after treatment, or if it is an unusual type, removal of the rectum and anus and creation of a colostomy may be necessary.

Each of the three primary treatments for anal cancer – radiation, chemotherapy, and surgery – has its own risks and possible side effects. Radiation treatments can cause blistering of the skin, fatigue, loss of appetite, possible loss of hair, diarrhea or constipation.

Common side effects of chemotherapy are:

- Nausea and vomiting
- Mouth sores
- Loss of appetite
- Hair loss
- Diarrhea
- Low blood counts

It's very common that chemo and radiation will begin simultaneously. I had a couple of weeks to prepare myself for the treatment. I've included a list that should be of help to you or your family member.

Follow-up care to assess the results of treatment and to check for recurrence is very important.

If you are not comfortable with the treatment plan your doctor has outlined for you, consider getting a second opinion. The emotional rollercoaster you may find yourself on during your diagnosis and treatment can be rather devastating. Having a strong support system will help during this time. If you don't belong to a church or have family and friends to help you, ask your doctor and the social workers at the hospital for suggestions.

While there is always the possibility of recurrence, treatments for anal cancer have some of the highest success rates when it comes to curing this dreaded disease, in part because if caught early the disease is confined to a relatively small area.

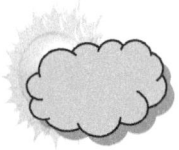 **Chapter 9: What to expect from week to week**

(Keep in mind that your experience will probably differ from mine.)

I'll share what happened to me and what you can expect in general. My understanding is that it's common protocol to start the chemo and radiation at the same time. Kind of a double whammy, but maybe it's good to get it all out of the way at the same time.

Week 1:

Day 1 (which was a Monday): Treatment started at the outpatient clinic where I had a Port placed. (A port is small medical appliance that is installed beneath the skin in which the chemotherapy drugs are administered.) This meant arriving 90 minutes before the procedure so the nurses would have time to prep me. Mine was placed in my right chest area just below the collar bone. For about a week I was sore from the port placement and had to be careful not to get it wet. You'll get instructions on how to care for it if you have this done.

Having a port was good idea for me because of all the blood work that has to be drawn and because of the type of chemotherapy I was given. We'll get to that in a bit.

Before you go to your port appointment find out if you're allergic to tape or bandages. They used a clear adhesive bandage to cover the port and it turned out that I was allergic to it. My skin is sensitive and it took about three months for the rash to go away.

Check with the nurses at the clinic and ask for a bandage that would normally be used for this procedure and put it on your skin for a little while to test to see if have a reaction. They do have another type they can use if you have a problem.

After I woke up from the port placement (yes, they give you what's called a conscious sedative) we went directly to the chemotherapy oncologist's office. First, I was given medication for nausea and then the nurse administered the chemotherapy meds. I was hooked up to a pump in a fanny pack that infuses the chemotherapy meds 24 hours per day for four days.

I was then given nausea medication to be taken for three days at home. This was enough to alleviate any possible occurrence of nausea and vomiting, which was a relief to me. What I did experience was a general feeling of yukkiness and I was queasy. I don't know how else to describe it.

Day 2: The day after chemo started I began radiation treatment. Since I'd already had an appointment the previous week to go through the orientation and positioning procedure, I knew what to expect. It's kind of weird, but my imagination is fertile and I had inaccurate images of how this was going to work.

There are no strange positions you have to get into. The radiation machine rotates to get in the correction position and radiate the area the radiologist has indicated.

These photos were taken after my radiation treatment was over. I asked the techs to take photos for this book to give you a visual image the position you're in.

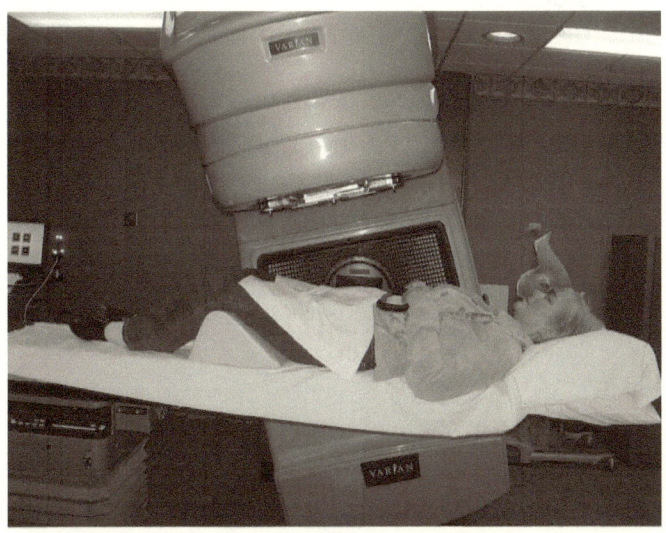

Radiation of pelvic area, top

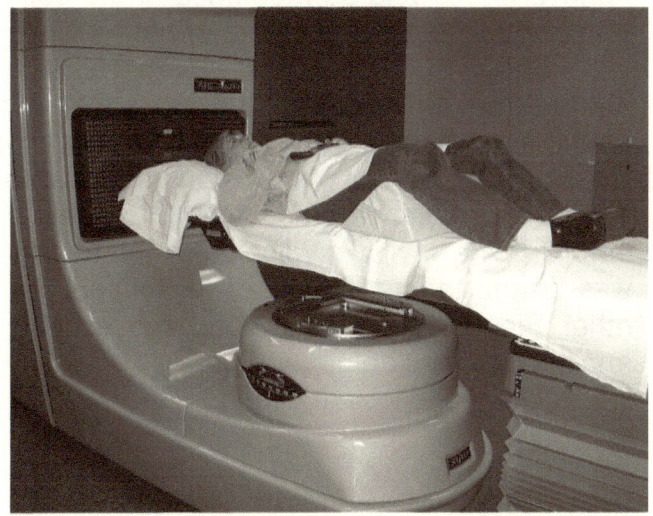

Radiation of pelvic area, bottom

The technicians were wonderful and very caring. I was scheduled at the same time every day. Radiation was scheduled five days a week with visits with the radiologist on Mondays. I also had appointments with the dietitian once a week to help me with my nutrition plan.

Radiation for this cancer can be anywhere from 17-30 treatments. It just depends on the individual and what the radiologist determines will be best for you.

Dealing with Stress:

My husband ordered a program for me called the Healing Codes. The Healing Codes were created to remove stress related memories at the cellular level, whether you're aware of them or not.

There are a series of hand positions that you hold for about 4-7 minutes 2 – 3 times a day. Doing the Healing Codes and my daily spiritual exercises helped keep me in balance emotionally. I did this every day before going in for my radiation treatments. Once I was on the table I imagined my spiritual teacher and other friends gathered around me singing HU (an ancient and holy name for God).

Day 3: I experienced queasiness, constipation, and difficulty sleeping. The latter was probably due to the discomfort of the newly acquired port. It hurt to turn over in bed.

I chose to take baths during this week to minimize the likelihood of getting the port wet. My husband washed my hair for me at the sink. This process got pretty old after awhile and I was very happy when I could again take a shower without worrying about getting the port wet. The reason for this is there's a higher chance of infection if water gets under the dressing.

After four days of the chemo pump I was more than happy to return it. Because it was a holiday when the pump was to be disconnected, the oncology doctor made an appointment for me at the emergency room to have an IV specialist deactivate the pump and remove the IV line. Normally, you'd go to your oncologist's office.

Spiritual Lessons I've Learned

The most important thing I've learned so far is that love is all there is. It's really the only thing that matters. If you have loved and been loved and can truly say you've brought joy to others, you've lived a good life.

It's just as important to accept love as to give it. How else can the people in our lives experience the gift of giving love?

Week 2 - 4:

After finishing eleven radiation treatments (out of 30) and one week of continuous chemo the side effects of chemo and radiation caught up with me.

It wasn't until the third week before I felt any pain or discomfort from the radiation. It's like having bad sunburn, only it's in an area that wouldn't normally be exposed to the sun, so it's even more sensitive.

Losing My Hair

I was running my fingers through my wet hair and came back with a handful of short salt and pepper hair in my hand. I thought it was feeling a bit thinner. A few days before I started chemo on Dec. 28th I had my hair cut short so that in case I did lose it, the baldness wouldn't be such a shock. Two and ½ weeks after chemo I started losing my hair. It's a good thing I have an extensive hat collection. I was shedding all over the place. As it turned out, I didn't lose all my hair, so I'm glad I didn't go ahead and shave my head as I was thinking I might.

Low White Blood Cells and Platelets

During week three I had my blood drawn and found out that my white blood cell and platelet counts were low. That means there's an increased risk of infection. My radiologist determined that I should take a break from radiation which coordinated nicely with my sore bottom. I wasn't sure how much more I could tolerate, to be honest. I finally gave in and started taking the pain medication she prescribed. Taking 1/2 of a pill every two hours seemed to work better than a whole pill every 4 hours. She suggested that I find the amount and timing that works best for me.

More Naps
Afternoon naps became part of my daily routine. I didn't seem to have a choice in this matter. Sometime around 2:30 pm my eyes started drooping and I couldn't stay awake. I took to having a snack and a nap just like when I was a kid.

Week 5:

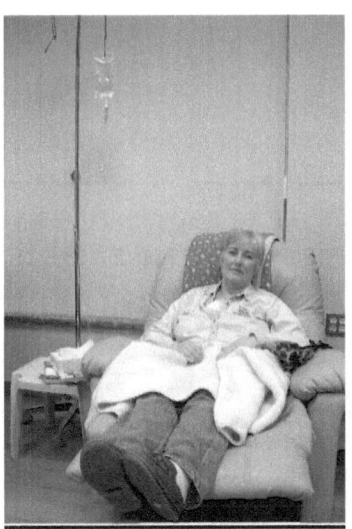

This time I know what to expect and it goes a little better than the first round.

I began the second round of chemo. Using earplugs at night helps to block out the every 30 second hum of the pump. Maybe some of you who have had this don't pay attention to it, but it can be annoying. I pretend it's singing HU (an ancient name for God) to me.

I did pretty well with the side effects, so far. The dietitian suggested that I start drinking a product called Juven. It has HGB, L-Glutamine and L-Arginine and helps promote wound heeling. It worked well for me as I only had to take ½ of a pain pill in the last week.

Pay Attention To Your Cravings

By paying attention to what your body is craving (within reason, of course) you may be able to give it what it needs nutritionally. The following is an excerpt from my blog journal:

Getting Over The Burn

"I've had about three weeks off from radiation treatment to allow my skin to heal. I won't go into the unpleasantries, but suffice it to say it's like receiving a severe burn and your skin peels. Ice packs and pain medication have been very helpful and create their own problems. It's just something you have to endure.

I am learning to listen to what my body needs. A couple of weeks ago when I had blood drawn at the oncologists office my platelets and red blood cell count was very low. There was talk of needing shots to increase the RBC's and platelets (at a cost of about $1,000 per shot). Just prior to learning what my lab results were, I told my husband that I was craving prime rib. That's very unusual for me since it's been 20 years since I've eaten red meat on a regular basis. When I asked the doctor what my other options were, she said to start eating red meat. Go figure!

Tuning into what my body is telling me has become increasingly important. I am learning to trust it and respond before being given a "doctor's order." There are so many lessons related to this illness and I'm really very grateful for all of them. That's what this life is about for me…learning who I am as Soul and giving and accepting God's love."

Drink Water Before Your Radiation Appointments

Pelvic radiation therapy always involves the intestines and bladder receiving radiation. Because of this, there is often abdominal cramping and diarrhea. The more you can protect the small intestine the better.

If you are able to hold a full bladder of urine, it is a good idea to drink as much water as possible 1/2 hour before your schedule treatment. This will help to move the small intestine up and out of the pelvis.

Because the vaginal area is being radiated, intense dryness and narrowing can occur and some doctors recommend vinegar and water douches as well as vaginal lubricants such as wheat germ oil. (Check with your doctor about this.)

Dealing with Constipation

My experience was different from the "norm". I was told that diarrhea is the more common side effect; however, I was constipated through the entire treatment. The following items are what I used to keep me regular.

Miralax
Hot water with lemon and honey
Stool softener
Senna tea

Keeping your digestive system as normal as possible will definitely be helpful during the last few weeks of radiation.

Dealing with Diarrhea

Diarrhea is a common side effect of radiation treatment (for anal or colon/rectal cancer).

I didn't have problems with diarrhea, but I did stock up on over the counter remedies for diarrhea just in case.

By the end of week five, I had to take a break from radiation which lasted almost three weeks. I was told at the beginning of treatment that I might have to take a break, but this was longer than expected.

Week 6:

This was my worst week. At the end of the fifth week the chemo pump was removed, but the side effects of the chemo drugs started sooner than they did with the first round.

I experienced thrush in the mouth, throat, and vagina: The radiologist prescribed Reynolds Solution. This was a life saver as it was even painful to drink water.

Severe pain with bowel movements: I used an ice pack on my bottom to numb it before I went to the bathroom and sitz baths afterward. I started using senna capsules and a stool softener, which did help.

Weeks 7 - 10:

I started back on radiation at the beginning of week 8.

Constipation was still a problem. It finally occurred to me that a cup of coffee might help with this. I drank a latte on the way home and had the desired effect. What a relief!

The rest of the treatment went ok. Of course there was pain and discomfort, but I was on the home stretch and seeing an end to treatment.

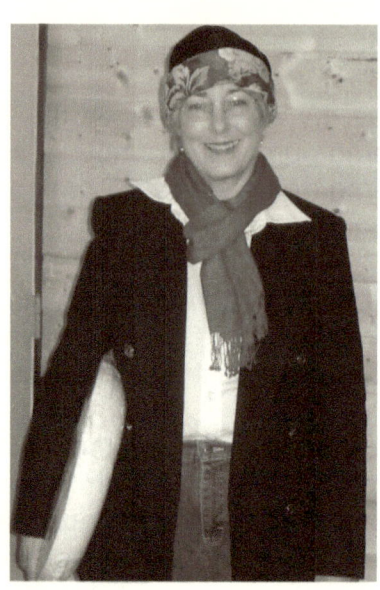

Week 8: Radiation begins again, so why am I smiling? Guess I know it will be over soon. My trusty donut goes with me everywhere.

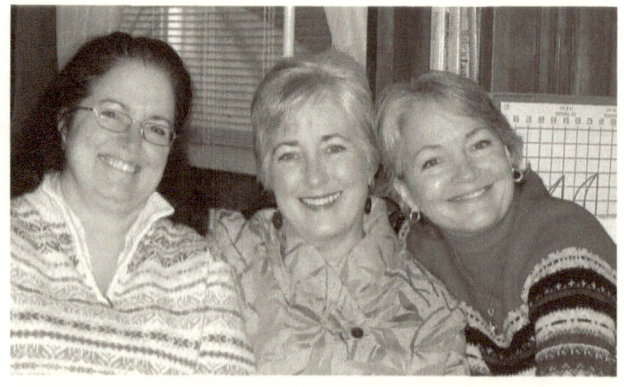

My sisters, (Jane on my left & Cecilia on my right) came to visit in January after my first round of chemo.

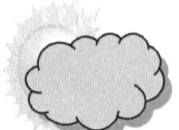 **Chapter 10: Stories and Experiences**

The following stories and experiences were contributed by several of my friends from www.BlogforaCure.com

Radiation and Deep Relaxation – by Nova Sprick

When I was going through radiation treatment three years ago, I wondered why the breast cancer ladies were in and out in a few minutes and I was lying on the table (in the frog position) for about 20-25 minutes each time. My radiology oncologist explained to me that I was getting "special" radiation…IMRT. As you might know this radiation is given from many different angles so as to try not to harm any one organ.

My doc suggested that I drink as much water as I could before treatment so I would have a full bladder and this also would help reduce unnecessary exposure to bowels.

The time on the table with all the great techs, actually became the best part of my day. I am a yogi and so, I would say a mantra (or prayer) as I entered the room asking that any fear that had been brought in by others be cleared from the room. Then I would get set up with a cd player on my chest and headset and begin playing Rod Stryker's Yoga Nidra tape. This is a form of deep relaxation that required you to set an intention rooted in gratitude and brings the body into a deep state of healing. I would also cover my eyes with an eye pillow and begin long slow deep breaths.

I was so relaxed that often I did not really want to get off the table. At first the techs thought I was nuts but then, when they saw how well I was doing they began to ask me if I had remembered to say my mantra and made sure my cd was all set at the proper start position.

For any of you who have gone through anal cancer radiation treatment, you know how burned you can get. I am very fair skinned but I have to tell you that I burned very little. Nothing like the other women I had seen…. I mean I was still wearing jeans at the end of my treatment….

I can't say for sure but I honestly believe that practicing Yoga Nidra each day was what allowed my skin to heal even as it was being burned….

Helpful Hints to Make Treatment Easier by Nancy

It does take time to heal like everyone else is saying. I too get impatient sometimes and think I am 9 months out of treatment and I still feel tired. Is there something wrong with me? Then everyone reminds me that I am doing so much better but that I can't expect to be back to normal so fast. My radiation doctor actually told me it would take 6 months to a year to feel anywhere normal. A couple things I might suggest:

1. Take time out for your family and friends. Life is definitely too short and as we all can see things can hit us when we least expect it.

2. Before I started radiation treatments my radiation doctor gave me a lotion to use everyday twice a day to get my skin moisturized before treatments even started. It was called "Special Care Cream". I could only purchase it at the hospital. Even though I did get burnt I think I would have been worse if I didn't use it.

3. I think women should know what radiation does to your vagina and how difficult it is to have sex. They should know to ask the doctors for dilators or where they can purchase them when treatment is over.

Suggestions from Daryl

1. I would emphasize the pain and do not sugar coat it...of course it is different for all of us...don't be afraid to load up on the pain meds!

2. Accept help from family and friends (this was extremely hard to do for me...I am very independent)...probably the hardest thing at all

3. It's ok to cry...many times while on the toilet I cried both from pain, fear and anxiety...it's a good release!

4. I was burned severely with radiation...although I knew it was happening I wasn't terribly vocal about it with the doc...this landed me in the hospital with an infection...if something doesn't feel right be vocal about it...although it is a standard treatment we are all different...I would emphasize that!

The following story is an excerpt from my blog.

Not-So-Ramdom Acts of Kindness by Theresa

God's love manifests in infinite ways and it's up to us to recognize it in our own lives.

During my illness and treatment for anal cancer that love has shown up as not-so-random acts of kindness committed by not only my friends and family, but also total strangers. I say "not-so-random" because I know that we are all vehicles for God's love. Spirit speaks to us all differently and sometimes in very subtle ways.

My sisters made plans immediately to come and be with us when they heard the news. It seems like a lifetime ago that they were here. They did things for me like making the slip cover for my sofa and driving me to my appointments. They were also very gracious in "letting" me cook and do things when I felt like it instead of insisting on doing everything themselves. There's a fine balance between being taken care of and doing things for yourself. They danced it with grace.

When my daughter, Jessie found out about my illness she was naturally very upset. She started crocheting a hat for me in case I lost my hair due to chemo. It didn't turn out exactly as she wanted so made a purse out of it instead. While at a Christmas party with her boyfriend's family, she made little cards with inspirational quotes on one side and hand drawn illustrations on the other. When everyone saw what she was doing they all joined in and created the most beautiful and unique gift I've received. I was so touched by the love I feel when I open that little pouch and think of all those wonderful Souls getting together to do something to help me feel better. I've never met any of them, yet hope to thank them in person.

My local friends call, send cards, and visit. A couple of them come out on a weekly basis to help me make applesauce or just visit. They also do energy work with me which has been so helpful. It brings a sense of peace and relaxation. What I find so endearing is that they're thanking me for letting them come and be of service in that way. Those are great friends!

Then there are my online friends from around the world. As a result of my online business ventures, I've met people from all over the world. When I told one friend from Australia about my illness, he asked permission to notify some of our mutual friends. It wasn't but a matter of a few hours before I started getting visits from several of them leaving comments on my blog to let me know that I'm in their thoughts.

One morning I was in the waiting room at the radiology office waiting to see the doctor. The lady next to me and I struck up a conversation. It turned out that she was driving her next door neighbor in for her radiation treatments a couple of times a week (that's a great neighbor!) and we happen to be neighbors ourselves. I have to mention that we live about 40 minutes out of town, so it was quite a coincidence (not). She was remarking on how much she liked the skirt I was wearing and I said that it was one of the most comfortable things I have to wear (because of where the cancer is located, skirts are the most convenient and comfortable clothing). She mentioned that she sews and could probably make another skirt for me just from using my skirt as a pattern. Mary Lee offered to go buy the fabric and have the skirt ready for me in a few days. My first inclination was to graciously decline, but the inner voice said to accept this gift of love. Now why is that so hard for many of us? Mary Lee came by with the new skirt, some home made chicken noodle soup and some home grown ground beef and sausage. She has a farm at the end of the road we live on. Her gifts so touched my heart. I hope you know people like her; the people in her life are truly blessed.

The staff at the radiology department where I received treatment were so good to me. They are friendly, understanding, and compassionate. I watched them with the other patients and it's the same for everyone they treat. For a short period of time we see these people on a daily basis and they become part of our lives. They are the only thing I miss about radiation treatment.

And then there's my husband, Hugh. His sense of humor, untiring patience with this process, and love has been my strength. He made sure I was always comfortable, taking care of the housekeeping, lots of the cooking, and our four-legged kids. He's the best husband anyone could dream of.

There are times I am so overwhelmed with the acts of kindness shown me that it brings me to tears.

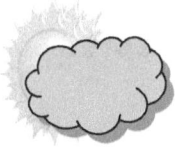 **Chapter 11: Support**

How to accept the love and help from family and friends

One of the lessons I've learned from this experience is how important it is to let the people in your life know how much you love them. I believe that's one of the biggest lessons we're here to learn; how to give and receive love.

So, the other side of it is receiving love. It seems like it's easy to do, but when it comes down to it how many times do I refuse help from people who care for me because I either don't want to be a burden or I don't want to give up my independence? It's important to allow other people the opportunity to give.

I received many calls and cards in the mail from friends and family. Sending warm thoughts of love is good and appreciated, but the actual phone calls, visits, and cards made a huge difference in how I healed.

We live in a physical world and need those tangible displays of affection. Let people do things for you even if you think you can still do it all for yourself.

If someone you are close to is going through an illness, your loving attention will be a blessing.

What to Say or Do for a Friend or Loved One Who Has Received the Diagnosis

The following suggestions are from my friends at Blog for a Cure:

"I sent Gemma (my grandmother) many a card even though we lived in the same house. The one that meant the most to her had a picture of two dogs (retrievers) swimming side by side and inside the card read, "I'm with you all the way." I think whatever you write, you should mean it and follow through."
Nancy G.

"When my daughter-in-law's mother was in the final days of her cancer struggle, in the hospital and no visitors, I had no idea what to write in a card. I finally wrote about some of the things she had accomplished in her life. Such as, "I was just thinking about how wonderful your daughters are. It must make you feel so good to know that you've raised such beautiful young ladies." Later, I was told that the card was placed in her casket with her."
Karen G.

"I like the idea of someone saying "thinking of you". I

was recently talking with a friend and realized that I didn't receive a bunch of cards when I was diagnosed… and it would have been nice to get some snail mail showing how someone is willing to take time out of their day and write to me their hopes that I get well…"
Grace

"Good to have this question. I agree that any sincere note, i.e. "You're in my thoughts and prayers." etc. is great. Anything that is well intentioned will always be well received. To NOT get anything from friends really hurts.

Offers of help, but specific ones… for example, someone offering to "help anytime, just ask" is nice but I'll never feel like I can call and ask for specific help. An offer like "I want to fix you dinner next week…how about Tuesday night?" Perfect. Or, "I know your son/daughter is going to the [insert function/game] here…I can take and/or drop them home…no problem."

Specific offers are really helpful.
Teresa

"Thinking of you is always good. At least you know they are. My husbands cousin has sent me a card every single week since the day I found out I was sick. Every one was different they always had some good scripture and she always ended her note with me and God love you. Her cards helped a lot. I have a couple of "friends" who hardly ever call any more. That is the toughest thing. What do they think, I'm contagious? Anyway it is nice to just get a card regardless of what it says." Eva

"For me, I have to have drivers to take me to appointments for when they put me under. It has been a godsend to have people volunteer to do that for me. I hate to ask anyone for anything.

I have a friend who has stage IV cancer and is about whipped. I would make dinners and drop them off at her husband's office in containers that did not need to be returned. Not only was she thankful, but her family was too." Kim

PART III - AFTER

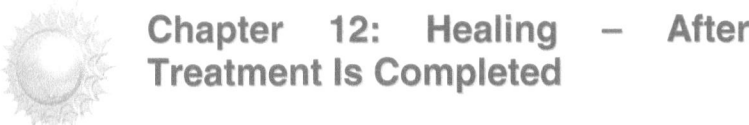 ## Chapter 12: Healing – After Treatment Is Completed

Follow Up Appointments

My oncologist and radiologist recommended that I see the surgeon about six weeks after the last radiation treatment. The reason for this is that the radiation continues to work for about that amount of time.

You'll probably be scheduled for follow-up visits every three to six months for several years to see if the cancer has recurred. This will also give you an opportunity to talk with your doctor about any side effects you may be experiencing.

So far, I've been having continued problems with constipation and have to experiment with different foods to find out what works best for me. You may benefit from talking with a registered dietitian or naturopathic doctor.

It's important to voice your concerns and symptoms so you get the help you need. This is not the time to be shy about how your body is functioning (or not functioning, if that's the case).

Possible Long Term Side Effects of Radiation:

- Frequent bowel movements
- Frequent urination
- Vaginal dryness
- Difficulty getting an erection

Vaginal Stenosis

Vaginal stenosis is perhaps the most long lasting and most difficult side effect of anal cancer radiation in addition to becoming menopausal if you are not already in this stage. For some the stenosis can be a serious problem. Stenosis is an abnormal narrowing of a tubular organ or structure.

Several weeks following completion of radiation treatment you may want to see your gynecologist about any scarring that has taken place and ask your doctor for vaginal dilators. There are several types and you'll need to find the one that works best for you.

In conjunction with your dilators, you may need vaginal jelly and you can talk about a prescription of Estradiol Cream.

One of the other concerns my radiologist had was that I might develop a fistula (from Wikipedia: an abnormal connection or passageway between two epithelium-lined organs that normally do not connect).

This was not the case for me; however, I pay attention to any changes in bowel function or vaginal discharge.

The following can be symptoms of a vaginal/anal fistula:

- Passage of gas, stool or pus from your vagina
- A foul-smelling vaginal discharge
- Recurrent vaginal or urinary tract infections
- Irritation or pain in the vulva, vagina and the area between your vagina and anus (perineum)
- Pain during sexual activity

Talk with your doctor if you have any of the above symptoms.

Lifestyle Changes

Now is the time to decide if you need and want to make some changes in your life regarding health, nutrition, exercise, emotions...lifestyle.

I always thought I was pretty healthy before my diagnosis, but I can see how more changes are necessary. It wasn't until I started doing the Healing Codes that I realized how much emotional baggage I was still hauling around with me. It's been a blessing to get rid of many of the beliefs about myself and others that no longer served me.

According to Carnegie Mellon University psychologist Sheldon Cohen and co-authors Denise Janicki-Deverts of Carnegie Mellon and Gregory E. Miller of the University of British Columbia, "Effects of stress on regulation of immune and inflammatory processes have the potential to influence depression, infectious, autoimmune, and coronary artery disease, and at least some (e.g., viral) cancers."

Eating Healthier

My eating habits were pretty good before cancer and now that I'm feeling better and can tolerate more fresh vegetables and fruit, I'll add them cautiously. Switching to organic is also something to consider. I believe moderation is still the key.

My mom was diabetic and it was suggested that she eat 5-6 small meals a day. This is something that works well for me because of the side effects to my digestive system. Working with a dietitian may help if you're having difficulty in this area.

Some suggestions are to cut down or eliminate all processed foods, change to organic fruits and vegetables, and reduce the amount of sugar, alcohol, and fats.

Getting Exercise & Rest

One of the effects of the radiation for me is being tired. It's different from the normal tiredness I experienced before the cancer diagnosis. This feels like pure exhaustion without a good reason for it.

Even though I often don't feel like going for a walk or doing any kind of exercise, this is actually something that will really help reduce fatigue.

Studies have shown that people who follow an exercise program feel physically and emotionally better and can cope more easily. Talk with your doctor before starting an exercise program, especially if you weren't very active prior to becoming ill.

Finding the right balance between activity and rest will come with experimentation. The first time I went for a walk after treatment was over I felt good enough to walk the same distance I had before treatment. I paid for it the next day by being exhausted and spending the entire day on the sofa. Pace yourself and you'll do much better.

Navigating Back To Self – by Nova Sprick from Blogforacure.com

"When we receive the diagnosis of cancer, it changes who we are, who we think we are, and how others see us. It is a transformation that affects us on all levels of body, mind and spirit. Unfortunately, the medical community is only trained to really treat us on a physical level and most people that are near to us want us to return to the same person we were before. However, our life is radically altered for at least some time if not forever.

Hopefully it changes us in a way that wakes us up to become even a bigger and better version of ourselves than existed before. This takes time, patience, commitment and fierce determination to want to change. It's hard, it's scary, and it asks us to push the boundaries. To let go of some things that no longer serve us (including relationships, food, lifestyle, jobs, etc. etc.). It means being totally honest with ourselves.

Most of us got anal cancer because we have HPV...so do a million other people. The problem is our immune system was not functioning optimally.

And the question to ask ourselves is why? While we need to let go of any blame we might place on ourselves, environment, or others, we need instead to turn our attention to making our life nurturing, fulfilling, honest, joyful, very healthy, and peaceful. This journey back to self begins right here...at home, within ourselves, and in the immediate world around us. It begins with the things we can control. We can look outside and see, smell, hear and taste pollution. All we can do is first look inside to create a clear, clean sparkling lake of the mind, body, heart and spirit within.

Navigating the new terrain of post cancer treatment is certainly a slippery slope. What works for one person doesn't necessarily work for another. But there are some things we can all do that will help us to find a way back to self or maybe even a more empowered self. What can we control? Well, we can surely choose a healthy lifestyle which includes diet (read Anti-Cancer Diet for Starters, exercise and yes, how we train our brains. The goal is to minimize stress on body, mind, and spirit and to emerge through self-advocacy, our own unique style of self-empowerment and with the help of support groups (whatever that means to you...a book group, family, this site, an organized cancer support group etc.) out of crisis and into wellness. Here are some things I found that helped me to realize my own beauty, strength, ability, and compassion once again.

1. **Breathe:** Most of us don't breathe fully. When we breathe from pelvic floor to up above our collar bones fully, a sense of calm fills our body quieting the nervous system and allowing our body to slow down to heal. There are so many

types of breath work but you can begin by lying on your back with a folded blanket under your ribs/chest/head; close your eyes...place your right hand on your low belly below your navel; practice breathing in this pelvic region. This area is shut down right now and by bringing breath to this area - feeling it expand on inhale and contract on exhale - we are creating a healing environment by providing good circulation here.

2. Then place your left hand on your middle belly and practice breathing in this area which is the healthy ego center and finally move your right hand up above the breast feeling your fingers spread from breath bone to collarbone and bring breath up here opening the heart. You can count with each breath...4 count inhale, 4 count exhale, repeating 'I'm breathing in love and healing," "I'm exhaling releasing all fear and toxins from my body, mind and heart." Then place your hands by your side and breathe from bottom to top in one long slow breath, pause, and exhale. Do this for 5 – 8 min a day

3. **Empower your self on a cellular level.** Write out a short script that you can memorize and easily repeat of how you see yourself, how you imagine or desire yourself to be. Example: I am a strong, healthy, vibrant and beautiful woman. My (husband, family, dog, partner etc.) adores me and sees me as strong, independent and vivacious. I show my husband every day how much I appreciate him. I'm good at what I do and I love my work. I feel so fit and healthy when I am out running etc. etc.), whatever it is that you see or want to see

yourself as. Say it as if it has already happened and repeat this script for at least 5 minutes each morning and feel it in the depth of your being until your cells believe it. If necessary go back later and try again.

4.   **Dance:** Move those hips. Sway your hips side to side, circle them (like jazz dancing). Take a belly dancing class if there is one in your area. Bring vitality back to your lower pelvis. Learn to love this area again! Put on music when you are cleaning and twist and turn, swing your hips.

5.   **Sit and quiet your mind.** Sit up on something (your knees should be lower than your groin). Close your eyes, envision your pelvis as a beautiful lotus flower and you a goddess rising out of the center. You can do this while you are doing step two or for another five minutes in the day. Repeat the mantra "I am healing every day; I am like a beautiful lotus flower rising out of the mud/muck and blooming into a serene, calm, and insightful goddess."

6.   **Put your feet up:** For 10 minutes (before bed is ideal) every day! Lay on the floor with your pelvis on a blanket about 4 or 6 inches away from a wall. Bring your legs up the wall and lay back, close your eyes. This pose is called Viparita Karani (look on yoga journal web site). Breathe long full breaths up the front of your body and down the back. Have some soothing music on and an eye pillow if you'd like. This will reverse the flow of blood, allow your lymphatic system to begin to circulate and move toxins out into the blood. It is also calming and you will sleep better.

7. **Get your lymph moving.** Start to detoxify by getting up and getting your lymph system moving in the morning. You can begin by a warm 3 minute shower; turn the water to cold for 1 minute and continue to alternate like this several times. Finish with warm of course, and then do a brisk self massage with some good warm body oil (sesame is preferred) moving in directions towards the heart working in back and forth strokes and circular strokes on joints, belly, and chest. You have lots of lymph nodes in your abdomen and feet, so be sure to spend time on these areas. Give yourself or ask your partner or friend to give you a good head massage with warm oil.

8. **Get a Massage.** Receiving is even better than giving one to yourself. Treat yourself; you will be amazed at how good you will feel.

9. **Soak.** Take a bath in bath salts with some nice essential oil dropped in...lavender for calming, peppermint for stimulating, rosemary for healing.

10. **Color your world:** Bring flowers into your house each week. Place some in family areas, some by your bed and in your bathroom. Wear colors. Buy some new clothes and wear purples and violet and blues and greens...all healing, and it will brighten you up. Be daring and wear color shadow on your eyes. Wear jewelry. If you are able to financially, get rid of the clothes you wore during treatment. These hold the energy you felt then. Otherwise, wash them several times. putting some lavender essential oil in the water.

11. **Keep a journal** and start writing out a list of those things that nourish you. Those things that make you feel sad, unworthy, unloved. Make a list of the qualities you admire in yourself and those that you wish to be rid of. Be honest. Make a dream board either real or in your mind of how you envision you will begin to live your life.

12. **Ask for what you need.**

13. **Let people know what you don't need.** I had a friend who would say to me "now you're a cancer girl too!" I do not think of myself as a cancer girl. I am Nova and I happened to have gotten cancer. It's gone and so I am not a cancer girl.

14. **Come up with your own ideas.** If you have always wanted red walls, but your family likes white, let them know that you want to create a space that is yours and reflects your own personality. If you don't know any more what you like, start finding that out. Look at magazines, read books, go on a weekend get away alone…begin to discover yourself.

For me learning to be really honest with what I need from life and love and family has been amazing. The more we learn to nourish our selves, our souls and hearts and minds; the more we ask for respect from others for our ideas, our thoughts etc., the more we will begin to attract health, love, and healing.

All of the above activities have allowed me to become stronger yet softer than ever (and I was pretty independent before). I am loved and more loveable than ever, more honest, freer, sillier, wiser, happier, healthier, and more compassionate. I hope you too will find them helpful. It takes great effort to do these things each day. But this is your journey now....a journey back to self.

Emotional Well-being

Now that treatment is over, you may feel unsure of what your routine and life is supposed to look like. There's been so much focus on getting through the treatment you may be confused about what's next.

This is when you will still need the support of your friends, family, church; whatever gives you comfort. It's been a turning point for me and many others to decide how to live the rest of our lives.

Cancer is now part of our story. We have the choice to move beyond it being the focus to making choices that will improve the quality of our life.

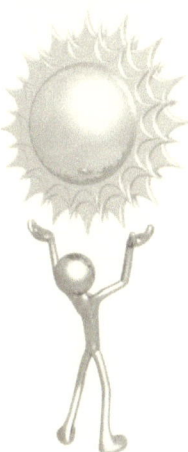

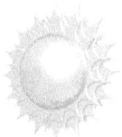 **Chapter 13 Thriving In Spite of Anal Cancer (or any other difficult situation)**

When something devastating happens (like getting the diagnosis of a potentially life threatening disease) it's understandable that we might ask, "Why me?"

The question I asked myself about my anal cancer diagnosis (after I had a little time to get over the shock) was, "What can I learn from this experience?" This was my key to thriving and growing spiritually during my illness.

Writing in my journal and my blog kept me from dwelling on the pain and discomfort so much. Instead, I paid attention to what I was learning about myself and the gratitude I felt for the love and gifts of time, food, cards, and phone calls from friends and family.

Remembering that I am Soul and I inhabit a physical body temporarily helps me keep all of my experiences in perspective. I am here to have experiences to teach me how to love . . . unconditionally.

5 Things That Help Me Thrive In Any Situation:

1. Count your blessings –Write down at least 3 things a day you are deeply grateful for.

2. Ask what you can learn from your experiences.

3. Do one thing for love every day. This means doing something for another that has no strings attached.

4. Accept the good will that comes your way. Instead of saying something like, "It's ok, I can do it myself." let other people help you. Giving and receiving go hand in hand . . . there can't be one without the other.

5. Daily contemplation or spiritual exercise – do whatever feels right for you regarding prayer, meditation, or contemplation. Spending time connecting to the Holy Spirit in whatever form you choose will help keep you in a more balanced state of consciousness.

About the Author

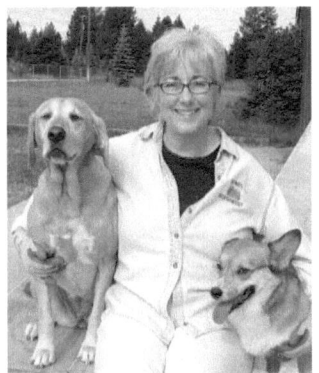

Theresa Mayhew is a spiritual student, wife, mother, semi-retired massage practitioner, writer, online entrepreneur and cleric. She and her husband, Hugh, their dogs Hunny and Maggi and four cats live on five acres in Elk, WA.

Her many interests include spending time with her husband, family and pets, sewing, reading, movies, creating websites, and spiritual studies. One of her favorite activities is being of service. She is active in her spiritual community of Eckankar, Religion of the Light and Sound of God.

Early in her massage career she volunteered many hours to the American Cancer Society's Relay for Life providing massage to the teams raising money and awareness for cancer never imagining that she would be directly affected by the illness.

In the six months since her last treatment for cancer, she has returned to the normal activities she enjoyed prior to being diagnosed. It took about eight weeks before she felt symptom free of the effects of radiation.

Theresa is back to her regular routine of working with her massage client, walking her two dogs, and has started a new business. You're warmly invited to visit her personal blog at TheresaMayhew.com

Life is good and she's enjoying every moment.

Resources

Blog for a Cure
This is a personal web publishing site for cancer survivors offering support. You'll find this to be a wonderful community of people who will support you during and after your treatment.

Cancer.org
The American Cancer Society is dedicated to eliminating cancer as a major health problem by preventing cancer, saving lives, and diminishing suffering through research, education, advocacy, and service.

National Cancer Institute – Cancer.gov
Accurate, up-to-date, and comprehensive cancer information from the U.S. government's principal agency for cancer research.

WebMD.com
Information on common types of cancer, including breast, lung, colon, skin, prostate, and ovarian cancer. Get the facts on cancer symptoms, treatments, and recovery.

Medicinenet.com
Learn about cancer types, disease statistics, facts, and survival rates.

HealthLine.com
This site provides relevant health information.

The Five Rites – These are physical exercises that resemble yoga. The book can be found at Amazon.com

The Healing Codes – You can get more information about this stress reduction program at StressManagementProgram.org

MindMovies – a program to create simple videos to help with visualization and goal setting. Example at TheresaMayhew.com

The Spiritual Exercises of ECK – discover how these spiritual practices can bring understanding, love, and balance to your life at Eckankar.org

www.ingramcontent.com/pod-product-compliance
Lightning Source LLC
Chambersburg PA
CBHW020400290526
45785CB00005B/2371